INTRODUCTION

How much time do you spend preparing to go to the gym? Most of us spend at least 15-30 mins just getting dressed and out the door.

Then, you likely drive 15 to 20 minutes to the closest gym. If you don't have a gym that is near you, your commute time may be even longer. You may be spending more time getting to the gym and back home than working out.

Once you get there, if someone else is using your favorite equipment, you may waste 10 or more minutes waiting for it to be free.

With all things considered, the gym can be quite time-consuming, costly, and draining.

However, the gym isn't your only option when it comes to staying in shape. Fitness doesn't have to be an all-consuming activity that forces you to take time out of your day to rearrange your schedule.

Right now, you might be thinking, *"If your goal is to lose weight, build muscle, or tone your body, then working out is essential."* **Yes, it is, but fortunately, you have other options than the gym, and can incorporate fitness tips right into your daily activities.**

"It takes about four days of virtuous living to create a little weight loss. That also happens to be the time required to get used to eating less.

In other words, if you can get past day three of a fitness regimen, things improve."

- Martha Beck

MOVE YOUR BODY

It's easy to get preoccupied with counting steps or repetitions at the gym. However, moving your body doesn't have to mean formal exercise. It's more time effective to focus on constantly moving your body instead of worrying if you're lifting enough weights or walking enough steps.

The key to staying in shape is constant movement.

When you get used to staying active all the time and finding new ways to move your body, exercise won't feel like a chore.

Keep these tips in mind throughout your daily routines:

1. **Learn to fidget more.** Do you move around in your chair? Do you play with the corners of your sweater or tug at your shirt? Fidgeting is often viewed in a negative way, but it can burn calories all day long. **Fidgeting can help you lose weight and stay in shape.** These small movements can add up to big changes in your body shape and weight.(don't look crazy though lol simple things to keep your body moving are key! Even if that means just staying busy at work)

- Feel free to swing your arms or legs, or simply tap your feet. You'll be burning calories. (when you go to the bathroom, get the most out of it!)

- Research studies support the idea of fidgeting more. One study from the Rochester Mayo Clinic in Minnesota found that fidgeting burns 54 percent more calories than being motionless or lying down.

- If you can fidget while walking, then you burn even more calories. The same study found that walking and fidgeting at the same time burned 154 percent more calories than being motionless.

- Your body is constantly burning calories. It's estimated that by simply sitting you can burn 600 calories a day. However, you can burn an additional 950 calories by fidgeting all the time. (Again, take this and incorporate it the best you can in your schedule)

2. **Find excuses to move more.** Whether you decide to walk around at the office during a break or stand up and move during a commercial on TV, the key is to keep moving.

    - Any time you're stuck waiting in an office or other location is a good excuse to get some exercise. You don't have to make it complicated. Simply walking or standing up is enough.

One of the best ways to incorporate fitness and exercise into your daily life is to move as often as possible and fidget frequently.

"My mother was a P.E. teacher, and she was kind of a fanatic about fitness and nutrition growing up, so it was ingrained in me at a young age.

As I get older, I'm finding out it's not about getting all buffed up and looking good [now]. It's more about staying healthy and flexible."

\- Josh Duhamel

CHANGE HOW YOU PARK

It's easy to get into a competition with another driver and battle for the best parking spot at the store or office.

But what if you changed how and where you park to add more fitness to your life?

Consider how much time you waste driving around a parking lot and looking for a space closer to the door. Then, consider that you could have spent less time by walking and probably finished your errands sooner.

The temptation to park as close as possible to the door isn't the best choice for your health or waistline.

Add more exercise to your parking routine with these strategies:

1. **Pick parking spots that are far away.** This goes against what you're used to

doing, but it's a smart way to add more fitness. Parking spots that are far from the door force you to walk more.

- You can get a great deal of exercise throughout your day by parking far away and walking.

2. **Deliberately take the long way back to your car.** Instead of looking for shortcuts, figure out how you can get more exercise.

    - By picking the longer route back to your vehicle, you'll get more steps and burn more calories. You can even walk around the parking lot a few times to get some extra fitness minutes.

Something as simple as parking far away can help you strengthen your heart and burn calories with ease.

"You need to put what you learn into practice and do it over and over again until it's a habit. I always say, 'Seeing is not believing. Doing is believing.'

There is a lot to learn about fitness, nutrition and emotions, but once you do, you can master them instead of them mastering you."

- Brett Hoebel

SWITCH TO A STANDING DESK

When you consider how much time you spend sitting at your desk at work or at home, you're losing a big opportunity to incorporate fitness into your routine. However, switching to a standing desk can help.

A standing desk forces you to be more active and burn calories. Researchers at the University of Pittsburgh discovered that you can burn an extra 8 to 10 calories for every hour you stand. Although this may not seem like a large amount, **it adds up over the course of a long work day.**

In addition, there are other advantages to using a standing desk, such as better posture, stronger muscles, and less back pain. Standing may also help you better regulate your blood sugar.

These tips will help you get the most advantages from using a standing desk:

1. **Keep moving.** Switching to a standing desk will help you immensely, but remember to keep moving as well. Flex your arms and tap your feet. Switch the positions of your feet.

    - **Alternate between sitting and standing.** Your legs will get tired if you're in front of a standing desk the entire day.

2. **Consider getting a treadmill-standing desk.** This is the ultimate way to work and exercise at the same time. A treadmill-standing desk forces you to run or walk all the time. Your body has to keep moving or fall off the treadmill.

3. **Follow the 20/8/2 rule.** This rule can help you get the most fitness out of your day while using a standing desk. The 20/8/2 rule refers to what you should do in each 30-minute time period.

- **During a 30-minute time period, sit for 20 minutes and stand for 8 minutes. Use the last 2 minutes to get up and move around.** This forces your body to keep moving and not get stuck.

- You can set an alarm at your desk to keep track of this rule.

4. **Focus on comfort.** One of the most important aspects when you switch to a standing desk is to remember comfort. You may spend eight or more hours at your desk. It's important to be comfortable while doing your work.

    - Buy shoes that are strong, yet supportive and comfortable.

    - Purchase an ergonomic or gel mat to stand on at your desk.

    - Also, you need a desk that's easy for you to use. If it's too hard, you'll soon get rid of it.

5. **Consider an adjustable standing desk.** The adjustments allow you to sit and stand at different intervals. An adjustable standing desk is more versatile and can be changed throughout the day or week to fit your needs.

Or, Alter Your Current Desk

Alternatively, if you can't, or don't want to, invest in a standing desk, you can try to adjust the one you have:

- Put your current desk on blocks to make it higher.

- Add books or plastic crates to raise your computer and keyboard, so you have to stand to reach them comfortably.

- You would still want to invest in a gel mat or other soft cushioning material for the floor because your feet will get tired from standing. It's important to consider the entire ergonomic situation of the desk.

Add more exercise to your life without going to the gym by getting a standing desk. You'll burn more calories and strengthen your health.

"I try to get seven hours of sleep every night; I always walk or bike to work; I make a point to eat well and take my vitamins; I drink tons of water; and I always spend a portion of my day at a standing desk."

- Jessica Scorpio

GET FIT IN YOUR COMMUTE

One of the best ways to add more fitness to your day is to change your commute.

If you're able to bike or walk to work, then the amount of exercise you can squeeze into your mornings may be enormous. Even if you're forced to drive or take public transportation, there are ways to add more exercise.

The key is to change how you approach your commute, so you can add a workout in the morning.

Consider these strategies to burn calories during your commute:

1. **Bike to work.** Many cities are committed to creating more green options and are offering more bike lanes. If your job is close enough, then consider switching to biking.

- Of course, biking is easier in warmer climates. However, even if you can only bike for a part of the year, you can make a big difference in your health.

- **Most experts recommend that you do not try to bike more than 30 or 40 minutes to work.** You're more likely to get tired and show up drenched in sweat if you go over 40 minutes of biking.

- You may need to pack an extra change of clothes if sweating is an issue while you bike. Also, consider the shoes you wear while you cycle. You can't do this in high heels or uncomfortable loafers. Pack shoes for the office and wear biking shoes.

- Some offices have welcoming policies for bikers and offer lockers or changing rooms. If your office doesn't have separate rooms for changing, you can change in the bathroom.

2. **Walk to work.** Walking is a good way to exercise in the morning if you live close to your job and can handle the commute on foot. Walking can burn 350 calories per hour.

    - **Experts recommend that you walk five or fewer miles to work.** Going over five miles is often difficult and can leave you exhausted before your work day has started.

    - Again, consider your clothing and shoes. You must wear comfortable footwear while walking, so you may need to carry an extra pair of shoes with you or keep one at work.

3. **Stand on public transportation.** If you take public transportation, you can still find a way to stay fit:

    - Standing instead of sitting on public transportation will burn more calories.

- Dance or move around during the stops. You don't want to do this while the train or bus is moving, but dancing or moving around is fine during a full stop. Avoid running into others or making a crowded space worse.

4. **Sing while you drive.** When your only option is to drive to work, getting exercise while you watch the road is trickier. You can't stand, and trying to fidget or move around while driving can put you and the other drivers at risk on the road. However, you can sing aloud while you're driving without hurting anyone.

    - Even if your voice is terrible, you can keep the windows up, so you're not annoying other drivers.

    - **Singing can burn 100 calories per hour while you sit.** If you have a long commute, then singing can help you burn calories in a safe way on the road.

5. **Take the scenic route to your office chair.** If your office has a courtyard or other natural spaces, take the scenic route before you sit down to work.

    - Some offices offer beautiful landscaping and courtyards. Take advantage of them by showing up to work early, so you can walk outside and enjoy nature while getting some exercise.

One of the best ways to add more exercise is to think of how you can change your morning commute. You can energize your entire day this way.

"The whole point of bike-sharing is to give New Yorkers another way to commute. A lot of folks in Bay Ridge work in downtown Brooklyn or other parts of the borough. For them, it would make more sense to hop on a Citi Bike [here] than to wait for a train or a bus [for work]."

- Sal Albanese

TAKE THE STAIRS

Taking the elevator is easier, but the stairs can help you stay fit. **The stairs are a better option for your health and waistline.** You may not be able to take them in every skyscraper, but you can make an effort to avoid the elevator.

Use these techniques to add the stairs to your daily routines:

1. **Choose the stairs.** Unless you're carrying a giant pile of papers or other heavy items that make walking difficult, the stairs are a better choice at work.

    - Each stair you climb burns 0.17 calories going up. You can burn 0.05 calories going down. The calorie amounts may not seem large at first, but they quickly add up if you climb several stories at a time, and do it more than once a day.

2. **Consider a strategy for tall buildings.** If you work in a skyscraper, it may not be possible for you to take the stairs all the way to your office. You'll get sweaty and tired before you even reach your desk. However, you can come up with a plan to tackle this dilemma.

    - Consider taking the elevator to a floor that is about two or three levels below your office. Then, take the stairs those last levels. This way you'll be able to get some exercise without being exhausted.

3. **Have a stairs buddy.** Some office stairwells are dark, lonely, and miserable. If you have a friend take the stairs with you, you'll avoid the loneliness of the area.

    - **You can also encourage each other to keep going as you climb the stairs.**

When you have the choice, pick the stairs. Your body and mind will thank you. In addition, you'll be getting some necessary exercise without rearranging your entire day.

"I'm an athlete, so I can get up one day and run and it wouldn't bother me. I don't get the time because I work for long hours every day. Being constantly on the move itself helps me stay fit. I don't go to a gym. I use the stairs, not the lift. I'm not into fitness, but I feel I should start, as it's healthy."

- Genelia D'Souza

MAKE PHONE CALLS COUNT

What if you started to look at phone calls in a different way? Most people sit down or stop walking when they're on the phone. However, if you're talking and not texting, you can still see what's around you and use this as an excuse to walk.

Researchers recommend that you use the opportunity to walk around each time you get a phone call. This will give you a short burst of energy and help you stay active.

Try these strategies to let the phone call you to action:

1. **Stand up or walk each time the phone rings.** When you have to answer the phone, use this as an excuse to move.
   - Think of the phone as your alarm to stand, even if the phone is right there on

your desk.

- Walk or continue to stand during the conversation.

2. **See the value in two minutes.** Most phone calls are short and don't last longer than two minutes, but they still have value.

    - **A study from the University of Utah School of Medicine found that two minutes of walking can counteract the dangers of sitting all day.** If you can walk for two minutes every hour, you can strengthen your health.

The phone can be your signal to get moving. It's an easy way to add some fitness into your routine.

"There are just some really beautiful people in the world. When you're walking down the street, or you're at a restaurant, someone catches your eye because they have their own look. It goes way beyond what they're wearing - into their mannerisms, the way they smile, or just the way they hold themselves."

- Mary-Kate Olsen

ADJUST MEETINGS AT WORK

How many times have you dreaded going to a meeting at work? You're usually stuck in a cramped room with a conference table, chairs, and technology. There's little space to walk around or move.

What if you adjusted how you handle meetings at work to incorporate more fitness?

Studies shows that employees are happier when they're able to move around and don't feel trapped in a conference room.

Use these strategies to make your meetings more physically and mentally beneficial:

1. **Switch to walking meetings.** You can walk around the office or take the meeting outside. A change of scenery can spark new ideas. Walking will also make you feel

more energetic

- Make physical activity a part of every meeting. You and everyone there will feel more alert and confident as you walk.

- The activity of a walking meeting can relieve stress and reduce pressure on those participating in the meeting. They may feel more comfortable and at ease, which encourages them to participate more fully.

2. **Consider having dedicated outdoor meetings.** Plan a weekly meeting in the courtyard, a local park, or nature center. Nature can soothe and relax you. Plus, by spending more time outdoors, you'll feel better and get more exercise without going to the gym.

The next time someone in your office wants to schedule a meeting, encourage them to have it outdoors or turn it into a walking meeting.

"Now, when an American has an idea, he directly seeks a second American to share it. If there be three, they elect a president and two secretaries. Given four, they name a keeper of records, and the office is ready for work; five, they convene a general meeting, and the club is fully constituted."

- Jules Verne

MOVE DURING YOUR LUNCH BREAK

How much exercise can you fit into your lunch break? From where you get your food to how you spend the break, you can make changes to get more exercise. Add to the fun and fitness by encouraging your coworkers to join you.

Try out these positive adjustments to get more activity during your lunch break:

1. **Get up from your desk.** It's easy to spend the entire day at your desk without moving or standing. The lunch break is your chance to get up and move.

    - Even if your only option is to eat in another room or walk around and go back to your desk, this is still an excellent opportunity to get moving. **Your body will appreciate every second of activity.**

2. **Get your food.** The best option is to keep your food in a fridge that's far away, so you'll have to walk to get to your food and you're not tempted to snack mindlessly. The extra steps to the fridge can add up during the week.

    - If you prefer to eat out during lunch, consider walking to a restaurant or café that is close to work. By walking, you'll burn calories and tone your legs.

3. **Use the break to run errands.** The lunch break is often the only chance you get to run errands. Consider how you can use the time to get more activities done. This is the time to catch up on tasks you can't do earlier or later in the day.

    - You may want to mail packages, pick up dry cleaning, or go shopping. Try to patronize shops close to your office so you can walk while running errands.

4. **Go outside.** If you're able to eat outside, use this opportunity to get fresh air and exercise.

    - During long lunch hours, consider walking or biking to a park to eat.

    - During short lunch hours, consider going outside to a courtyard near your office or simply outside your building.

    - Even if you don't have a dedicated green space near your job, you can still enjoy the fresh air. You may be able to find a quiet balcony, sidewalk, or other nook that gives you room to pace.

5. **Get a workout.** If you can squeeze in a workout during lunch hour, this is ideal. You can do short workouts in your office or outside in the fresh air. Organize your coworkers to form a small team of dedicated exercise partners.

- Use the time to practice yoga, do aerobics, or even play a friendly game of sports.

Exercise can become a normal part of your lunch break at work. You may even look forward to it every day.

"When I produce a movie - and I've produced a number of movies, unlike Arnold - yes, I'm frustrated when the union says you can't do this, you can't work past that hour, you've got to break for lunch. But ultimately, they're right [about it]. What they do is [really] for everyone's benefit."

- Warren Beatty

EXERCISE WHILE WATCHING TV

TV can absorb a great deal of your day or evening, but are you using the opportunity to add exercise and avoid being a couch potato?

Simply adjust your TV routine to add some light exercises, like this:

1. **Start by exercising during commercials.** If you're used to just sitting, it may be hard to jump right into working out while watching TV. You can start by doing light exercises or movements during commercial breaks, such as walking around the room.

    - Since there are multiple commercials in one hour, you'll be surprised by how much activity you can squeeze into TV time.

    - As you get more used to being active, add small workouts like lifting weights or jogging in place. Another option is to do yoga or aerobics.

2. **Turn it into a game.** Have fun with exercise while you're watching TV! Consider doing a jumping jack each time your favorite character does something funny or stand up each time the villain comes on the screen.

    - This will encourage you to keep moving and look forward to the action on the screen, so you can do your own version at home.

3. **Keep snacks far away.** If you bring snacks to the TV area ahead of time, not only will you be tempted to overeat, but you'll also be losing out on the chance to move to go get them.

    - Walk to the kitchen each time you need a refill or more food. This will force you to reconsider your food choices and make you exercise at the same time.

4. **Move exercise equipment to the TV room.** Where do you keep your treadmill? Avoid leaving your exercise equipment in a corner of a room you rarely use. Instead, put it in front of the TV.

    - You'll be able to work out and watch your favorite shows at the same time. You'll be more motivated to exercise.

    - Many people complain about how boring exercise can be at home. However, watching TV can make it fun. You may be surprised by how many miles you can run on the treadmill as you watch an action show.

5. **Compete with others.** If you're lucky to watch TV with friends or family, then turn it into a workout competition.

    - How many pushups can you do compared to your friend while the commercial is on? How many jumping jacks can you both do during a break? **The key is to make the competition fun and easy.**

- You can create rewards for the winners that range from silly things to serious items. For example, one reward can be getting to choose the next show you watch together.

6. **Do simple chores.** When you're watching TV, you can still pay attention to the show while doing some chores that burn calories.

    - Use your arm muscles and fold laundry.

    - Sweep, mop, or dust the room.

7. **Create an obstacle course in front of the TV.** Circuit training and obstacle courses are popular at gyms, but you don't have to go to the gym to benefit from obstacle courses. Create your own in front of the TV.

- Rearrange furniture and pillows to make a simple course.

- You can also use laundry baskets, plastic tubs, or other items.

TV time doesn't have to mean eating chips or candy while zoning out on the couch. You can use this time to exercise, get in shape, and make an active lifestyle a normal part of your routine. Make losing weight fun when you make it a part of watching TV.

"Most people just half-watch TV. They watch TV while they are doing many other things in the environment of their home. So, what they are doing goes through their ears as much as through their eyes. In television, the narrative and characters are in the foreground of everything, because you are watching TV as you do other stuff."

- Alfonso Cuaron

CHANGE HOW YOU SHOP

How many hours do you spend every month buying food and other items? Are you using these hours to their fullest extent when it comes to exercise, fitness, and staying active? When you consider how much of your week is spent shopping, you may want to adjust how you handle this activity.

Change your shopping habits to add more fitness:

1. **Use baskets instead of carts.** Unless you're buying bulky items that weigh too much, consider using baskets instead of carts. **Baskets force you to use your arms and other muscles to carry the items you pick out.**

2. **Shop in the real world.** Shopping online usually means you're sitting at a desk or on the couch. **Shopping in the real world forces you to walk and use your body.** All of the activities of physical shopping add

up, especially if you hit more than one store in each trip.

3. **Go around the perimeter of the store.** Even if your items are in one spot, you can get a good workout by taking the time to walk around the entire shop.

    - You'll burn calories as you walk from aisle to aisle. You'll be entertained by watching other shoppers and looking at the items, so you may not even notice the exercise.

4. **Try mallercise.** "Mallercise" is short for mall exercise. You may see groups of people walking together at your local mall. Power walking is quite popular. Some malls even open early to allow people to walk in the mall.

    - Senior citizens aren't the only ones who get involved. You can start your own mallercise group and get active while you shop.

5. **Carry your bags.** You can get a workout by carrying your own bags. The bags are like weights and help you tone your body. They'll help you get in shape and stay that way.

Shopping can be a fun way to exercise and move your body!

"Yes, e-commerce is a strange situation for an old guy like me. You can buy a TV online, OK, but to buy a dress or shoes? Ugh. The customer has to go back to the store and breathe and smell and have a good time. Because shopping is a good time - like going to a nice restaurant."

- Max Azria

USE FITNESS TRACKERS

Fitness trackers can motivate you to get moving and stay in shape.

A study from the National Institutes of Health found that the self-monitoring created by using fitness trackers is beneficial. **Researchers also found that a fitness tracker could make you more likely to make significant lifestyle changes that strengthen your health.**

See how a fitness tracker could benefit you:

1. **Track your progress.** One of the main benefits of using fitness trackers is to ensure you're making progress.

    - A fitness tracker can show you the total number of steps you walk and the calories you burn. It can also show your heart rate, pulse, and other body data.

- **Researchers point out that what gets measured is more likely to be managed.** This means that you're more likely to change or pay attention to things that you're tracking and measuring. Attaching numbers to things can raise their significance in your mind.

2. **Increase your motivation.** When you see the number of steps you've walked since morning, you're motivated to keep going.

    - You may notice you want to exercise more because you're wearing a fitness tracker.

    - It can serve as a constant reminder that something is monitoring your activity levels.

    - Sometimes simply seeing a low number on the tracker can encourage you to move.

Fitness trackers are a convenient way to ensure you're getting enough exercise and know that it's making a difference. There are many types of fitness trackers. Comparing various trackers in your price range will help you pick out one that will work well for you.

"Staying more controlled mentally stemmed from taking my fitness more seriously. When you're doing track work, sprints and so on, it's pretty painful, but that does make you feel better prepared and therefore mentally stronger when you're going into a match. You know, without a doubt, that you are strong enough to last."

- Andy Murray

DO MORE YARD WORK

Instead of paying someone else to maintain your yard, consider how you can use this as an opportunity to burn calories. **Yard work is a rewarding way to incorporate fitness into your daily life.**

From mowing the lawn to pulling weeds, you can get a complete workout while making your yard beautiful.

Try these activities:

1. **Grow a garden.** One of the most rewarding ways to get more fitness into your routine is to start a garden.

    - A garden requires regular and ongoing maintenance. You'll have to take care of it, if you want it to survive. This may mean weekly chores to keep it alive.

- Gardening can range from growing a few flowers to filling your fridge with all the vegetables your family can eat. **The key is to find a happy balance that keeps you active and motivated to work in the garden.**

- From raking leaves to adding more soil, you'll find many activities to keep you busy.

2. **Pull up all the weeds.** Instead of spraying chemicals, consider doing this the old-fashioned way. Pulling out weeds can be a great workout. Each time you see a weed, stop and remove it. This will always keep you active and moving.

3. **Use a push mower.** If you want a major workout, then get a push mower to cut the grass in your yard. It's a heartier fitness choice than riding mowers.

- Your heart rate will increase with a push mower, and you'll burn more calories.

4. **Make watering a chore.** Use a hose instead of sprinklers. You'll have to drag a heavy hose around the yard to water everything, so your arms will get a work out.

5. **Rake leaves.** Avoid using a blower to collect the leaves. Instead, use a traditional rake and get your whole body active.

6. **Use a wheelbarrow.** Wheelbarrows can help you haul waste and other items in the yard. They tend to be heavy, so your muscles will be forced to stretch and move.

    - You can also use the wheelbarrow as an exercise tool and take multiple loops around the yard or garden.

The next time you notice weeds in the yard or the grass getting too high, don't call the maintenance crew. Instead, do it yourself and get the benefits of exercise.

"Exercise, from a public health perspective, is an unmitigated failure. The world's longest-lived people live in environments that nudge them into more movement. They don't use power tools, they do their own yard work, they grow a garden. Walking is the only way proven to stave off cognitive decline – it works."

- Dan Buettner

DANCE

One of the reasons people avoid the gym is because they find the routine boring. A good alternative is dancing. Dancing is a powerful way to exercise, tone the body, and lose weight.

Take advantage of dancing to drop those extra calories:

1. **Add dancing after dinner.** When you're going out to dinner, pick a restaurant that has dancing. Dancing after dinner can burn the extra calories you consume.

2. **Sign up for a dance class.** When going to the gym makes you want to cry, consider giving dance a chance. It's more fun and has better music.

    - Dance classes can be done one on one or in group settings.

- You can pick the music and genre that you love.

3. **Dance at home.** You don't need a class to move your body. You can dance at home in front of the TV or dog. You can get dance videos online or other locations and learn new moves. You can practice without worrying about judgment.

4. **Dance while you cook.** You're about to eat more calories, so dancing while you prepare the food is a wise choice. Consider dancing while you get ingredients together, stir things, or wait for the food to cook.

5. **Dance as you get dressed.** Turn your regular routine into a fun dance. Add dancing to your dressing ritual. You can make each part of your outfit into a different move.

Dancing is a fun way to move the body and stay active. Moving to music can make you forget that you're getting a serious workout.

"I've always believed fitness is an entry point to help you build that happier, healthier life. When your health is strong, you're capable of taking risks. You'll feel more confident to ask for the promotion. You'll have more energy to be a better mom. You'll feel more deserving of love."

\- Jillian Michaels

CONCLUSION

What if you didn't have to go to the gym all the time and could still benefit from exercising?

You don't have to commit to difficult exercise routines or long hours at the gym to see changes in your body. There are easy ways to incorporate more movement and fitness into your daily routine, so you burn calories, stay in shape, and strengthen your health.

Incorporating fitness into your daily routines is the key. You get all the health benefits without the exercise feeling like a tedious chore.

Consider your typical daily routine and ways you can adjust it to be more active. Can you go for a walk in the park? Can you take the stairs instead of the elevator? Consider changing how you shop, work, play, and watch TV. From walking to work to parking far away, you can make small changes that matter.

When you look at your day, you'll see opportunities to move more. **You may struggle with the changes at first, but they'll become easier over time.**

Look forward to exercise instead of dreading it. There's a reason why so many gym memberships fail, and it's related to how you think about fitness. Making exercise a normal part of your day will change your outlook and allow you to enjoy being fit – maybe for the first time!

www.ingramcontent.com/pod-product-compliance
Ingram Content Group UK Ltd.
Pitfield, Milton Keynes, MK11 3LW, UK
UKHW060405300726
14090UKWH00006B/452

* 9 7 9 8 4 1 9 5 0 0 3 6 5 *